INTEGRATIVE ONCOLOGY APPROACHES

A Complete Guide For Unveiling Hope And Bridging Paths For Empowering Healing

WALTER ZYAIRE

DISCLAIMER

The information in this book is intended only for general informational purposes; it should not be used in lieu of professional advice or medical care. Since the author is not licensed to practice therapy, the information offered should not be used in place of the expertise, judgment, or guidance of qualified mental health or medical professionals. Readers are encouraged to consult therapists, medical specialists, or other qualified authorities regarding their particular situation and needs. The publisher and author disclaim all liability for any actions or decisions taken by readers based on the information in this book. Results may vary from person to person and this book's approaches, procedures, and strategies may not be suitable in all circumstances. Considering unique situations and consulting a qualified expert are essential when choosing the right course of action. Neither the publisher nor the author recommend or guarantee the efficacy of any therapy or treatment that is indicated in this book. Because the information is based on the author's research and understanding at the time of publishing, it could not reflect the most recent developments or practices in the treatment area. The publisher and the author both disclaim all liability for the accuracy, completeness, or use of the material in this book. Readers bear full responsibility for the decisions and actions they choose in light of the information presented in this book.

TABLE OF CONTENTS

ABOUT THE BOOK

The book "Integrative Oncology Approaches" is very important when it comes to cancer therapy and care. It offers a broad perspective that transcends conventional cancer treatments through its thorough investigation of integrative approaches to oncology. The groundwork is laid in the introductory chapters, which emphasize the importance of holistic cancer care and the need for an all-encompassing strategy to handle the disease's intricacies.

The book provide readers with a thorough understanding of the framework in which integrative approaches function by delving into the principles of cancer biology, various forms of cancer, and the stages and grades of the disease. An understanding of conventional cancer treatments, such as immunotherapy, radiation therapy, chemotherapy, and surgery, is essential before moving on to the topic of integrative techniques.

The merger of conventional and integrative medicine is examined in the book's last chapters, with a focus on patient education and empowerment, possibilities, and problems for medical professionals to work together on. "Integrative Oncology Approaches" is a great resource for cancer patients, healthcare workers, and anybody else looking for a thorough understanding of integrative tactics in cancer care because of its collaborative and holistic approach.

The introduction of integrated methods to can
is the central feature of the book. In this part
misconceptions and myths about integrative c
are debunked as the fundamentals of the f
defined and outlined. Subsequently, the book
into distinct integrative methods, including
adjustments, mind-body strategies, nu
approaches, and complementary therapies, all
are covered in separate chapters. The focus or
modifications, stress management, and diet h
the complexity of cancer care.

The book offers focused insights on in
strategies for particular cancer types, ackno
the particular difficulties and factors associa
each. The book discusses quality of
survivorship. It provides advice on what to
cancer treatment, how to deal with long-t
effects, and how to maintain mental and c
health.

The introduction of integrated methods to cancer care is the central feature of the book. In this part, typical misconceptions and myths about integrative oncology are debunked as the fundamentals of the field are defined and outlined. Subsequently, the book delves into distinct integrative methods, including lifestyle adjustments, mind-body strategies, nutritional approaches, and complementary therapies, all of which are covered in separate chapters. The focus on lifestyle modifications, stress management, and diet highlights the complexity of cancer care.

The book offers focused insights on integrative strategies for particular cancer types, acknowledging the particular difficulties and factors associated with each. The book discusses quality of life and survivorship. It provides advice on what to do after cancer treatment, how to deal with long-term side effects, and how to maintain mental and emotional health.

The merger of conventional and integrative medicine is examined in the book's last chapters, with a focus on patient education and empowerment, possibilities, and problems for medical professionals to work together on. "Integrative Oncology Approaches" is a great resource for cancer patients, healthcare workers, and anybody else looking for a thorough understanding of integrative tactics in cancer care because of its collaborative and holistic approach.

CHAPTER ONE

OVERVIEW OF INTEGRATIVE ONCOLOGY APPROACHES

INTEGRATIVE ONCOLOGY OVERVIEW

Integrative Oncology is a more patient-centered and comprehensive approach that has revolutionized the field of oncology in recent years. To address the physical, mental, and spiritual aspects of the disease, this holistic approach emphasizes the integration of conventional medical treatments with alternative therapies, acknowledging the complex character of cancer. Integrative oncology recognizes the value of treating the patient as a whole, not just the tumor, which extends beyond the parameters of the conventional cancer care paradigm. This strategy seeks to improve cancer patients' quality of life and general well-being throughout their therapy.

The multidisciplinary discipline of integrative oncology blends complementary medicines, lifestyle modifications, and mind-body techniques with evidence-based traditional cancer treatments. The objective is to maximize patient outcomes by addressing the various facets of cancer and how it affects a person's life. This method recognizes the connection between a person's total health and several interrelated aspects, including lifestyle, psychological factors, and heredity. Integrative Oncology seeks to develop a more individualized and customized approach to cancer therapy by incorporating these variables into the treatment strategy.

 The use of complementary therapies, including as acupuncture, massage, nutritional therapy, and mind-body practices like yoga and meditation, is a crucial component of integrative oncology. These treatments were selected because they can lessen the negative effects of cancer treatments, help patients manage their symptoms better, and improve their general quality of life. Scientific evidence and a patient-centered approach direct the integration of these therapies, guaranteeing the safety and efficacy of interventions.

THE VALUE OF COMPREHENSIVE CANCER TREATMENT

Integrative Oncology's emphasis on holistic cancer care highlights the importance of treating the patient as a whole rather than just the disease. In addition to its physical effects, cancer is a complicated illness with significant emotional and psychological ramifications. Recognizing the interdependence of these elements, holistic cancer care attempts to offer patients receiving a cancer diagnosis all-encompassing support.

Incorporating holistic approaches into cancer care entails taking into account the patient's social support networks, lifestyle choices, mental and emotional health, and the tumor itself. Studies have indicated that a comprehensive strategy can help cancer patients adhere to their treatment regimens more closely, experience less stress, and have a higher quality of life. Holistic cancer care acknowledges and addresses the larger parts of a patient's experience to enable them to take an active role in their recovery.

Integrative oncology is a forward-thinking, patient-focused method of treating cancer that combines traditional medicine with complementary therapies. Holistic cancer care emphasizes treating the patient as a whole, recognizing the complex relationship between physical, emotional, and spiritual health. By adhering to these values, Integrative Oncology hopes to improve the general quality of life for those who receive a cancer diagnosis and open the door for a more individualized and all-encompassing approach to cancer treatment.

CHAPTER TWO

COMPREHENDING CANCER

FUNDAMENTALS OF BIOLOGICAL CARCINOGENESIS

A thorough understanding of cancer biology is necessary, as aberrant cellular proliferation upsets the delicate equilibrium of the body's regulatory systems. Fundamentally, cancer is a collection of disorders marked by unchecked cell proliferation and division, which results in the development of malignant tumors. These tumors pose a serious risk to general health because they can spread to other parts of the body and infiltrate nearby tissues.

Understanding the typical mechanisms of cell growth and division is essential to understanding the fundamentals of cancer biology. To preserve tissue integrity, cells must replicate and divide in an orderly fashion, which is ensured by the closely controlled cell cycle.

Cancer develops when a cell's DNA is mutated to interfere with this regulatory system, enabling the cell to escape typical growth constraints. Numerous things, including as genetic predisposition, exposure to carcinogens, and mistakes made during DNA replication, might result in these mutations.

VARIOUS CANCER TYPES

It's important to acknowledge the wide range of cancer kinds that exist in addition to the broad understanding of cancer. Cancer is a group of diseases with various characteristics rather than a single illness. Sarcomas develop from connective tissues such as muscles and bones, whereas carcinomas, the most common kind, originate from epithelial tissues.

While lymphomas affect the lymphatic system, leukemias impact the bone marrow and blood. Comprehending the many categories is essential for precise diagnosis, prognosis, and therapy strategizing.

CANCER STAGES AND GRADING

A key factor in assessing the scope and gravity of the illness is the cancer's stages and grading. Assessing the tumor's size, the extent of invasion into neighboring tissues, and the likelihood of metastasis to lymph nodes or other organs are all part of the staging process. Clinicians can forecast the prognosis and choose the best course of treatment with the use of this information. Grading, on the other hand, evaluates how aberrant cancer cells are in comparison to healthy cells. Higher-grade tumors may need more extensive therapies and frequently exhibit more aggressive behavior.

The various forms of cancer are diagnosed using different staging and grading methods. The TNM technique, which is frequently applied to solid tumors, evaluates the main tumor's size and extent (T), the involvement of neighboring lymph nodes (N), and the existence of distant metastases (M). Together, these variables influence the cancer's overall stage.

Grading, which is commonly represented as well-differentiated to poorly differentiated or G1 to G3, offers more information about the cellular makeup and behavior of the tumor.

A thorough comprehension of cancer necessitates exploring the complex processes of cancer biology, identifying the various forms of the disease, and appreciating the role that stages and grades play in defining how the illness progresses. The intricacies of cancer are still being uncovered by research, which directs the creation of more specialized and potent treatment approaches to tackle this complicated group of illnesses.

CHAPTER THREE

CONVENTIONAL CANCER THERAPIES

OPERATION

The mainstay of conventional cancer treatment is surgery, which is frequently used to remove tumors and the tissues around them. Surgery's main objective is to remove malignant growths that are localized and haven't spread far. Surgeons have access to a variety of tools, including minimally invasive treatments like laparoscopy and open surgery. Surgery by itself might be curative in some circumstances, particularly if the cancer is localized and found early. To maximize its efficacy and target any residual cancer cells, surgery is commonly paired with additional forms of treatment like chemotherapy or radiation therapy.

CHEMOTHERAPY

Another essential part of conventional cancer treatment is chemotherapy, which uses medications to either kill or stop the growth of cancer cells. These medications can be injected or taken orally, and they work by traveling throughout the body to target the main tumor as well as any possible metastases. Chemotherapy is a systemic treatment, meaning that it affects every region of the body; nevertheless, it is especially helpful when the cancer has spread or when metastasis is highly likely. Chemotherapy is an effective treatment, but because it affects normal cells that divide quickly, like those in the bone marrow and digestive system, it frequently causes a variety of side effects. Targeted medicines have advanced to specifically target cancer cells to reduce these negative effects.

RADIATION TREATMENT

High doses of ionizing radiation are used in radiation therapy to harm or kill cancer cells. This is a targeted treatment that goes after particular regions where tumors are found. Radiation can be injected internally by putting radioactive materials inside the tumor or externally by using devices like linear accelerators. The goal is to cause damage to the cancer cell's DNA so that it stops it from proliferating and dividing. For some tumors, radiation therapy is frequently used either alone or in combination with chemotherapy and surgery. Radiation therapy may have side effects, mostly in the surrounding healthy tissues, but advances in technology and treatment planning have increased accuracy and reduced collateral damage.

IMMUNOTHERAPY

Using the body's immune system to identify and combat cancer cells, immunotherapy is a relatively new concept in cancer treatment. Immunotherapy strengthens the body's defenses against cancer, in contrast to conventional treatments that attack cancer cells directly. Several strategies are used, including therapeutic vaccinations, adoptive cell therapy, and immune checkpoint inhibitors. For example, immune checkpoint inhibitors prevent immunological responses by blocking proteins, which improves the immune system's ability to identify and combat cancer cells. Research is currently being conducted to increase the applications and enhance the efficacy of immunotherapy for a wider range of cancer types, as it has demonstrated extraordinary success in treating several malignancies. Immunotherapy does not, however, work for every patient, and for best outcomes, it may be combined with other conventional treatments.

CHAPTER FOUR

COMPREHENSIVE METHODS FOR CANCER TREATMENT

INTEGRATIVE ONCOLOGY'S DEFINITION AND GUIDING CONCEPTS

Integrative oncology is a complete approach to cancer therapy that addresses the physical, emotional, and spiritual elements of a patient's well-being by combining alternative therapies with standard medical treatments. Integrating evidence-based complementary medicines with mainstream cancer treatments while maintaining a patient-centered approach is the key idea. This approach seeks to improve the overall quality of life for cancer patients while acknowledging that cancer care goes beyond the disease itself.

A multidisciplinary team of healthcare providers, comprising medical oncologists, naturopathic physicians, dietitians, mental health specialists, and other complementary practitioners, collaborate by the fundamental tenets of integrative oncology. Treatment regimens are tailored to each patient's specific requirements, taking into account personal preferences, general health, and the kind and stage of the cancer.

The goal of integrating alternative and conventional therapies is to maximize therapeutic benefits while reducing adverse effects and enhancing the general health of the patient.

INTEGRATIVE MEDICINE'S ADVANTAGES IN THE TREATMENT OF CANCER

Regarding cancer treatment, integrative medicine has several advantages. Enhancing the effectiveness of traditional therapies like radiation therapy, chemotherapy, and surgery is one major benefit. Acupuncture, massage, and mind-body techniques are examples of complementary therapies that can assist control adverse effects associated with treatment, reduce pain, and enhance treatment tolerance in general.

Integrative medicine places significant emphasis on the holistic well-being of its patients. Integrative approaches to cancer care include psychological and emotional factors in addition to the physical. Counseling, support groups, and mindfulness-based stress reduction can all help with mental health and emotional resilience—two essential elements of overcoming a cancer diagnosis.

Furthermore, integrative medicine places a strong emphasis on lifestyle elements like sleep, exercise, and nutrition since it understands how they affect the immune system and general health. Integrative methods encourage patients to take an active role in their recovery by giving them a sense of agency and self-efficacy.

TYPICAL MYTHS AND MISCONCEPTIONS

There are still misunderstandings and misconceptions about integrative oncology, despite its increasing recognition.

An often-held misperception is that integrative therapies are complementary approaches intended to supplement traditional cancer treatments. In actuality, integrative medicine enhances conventional therapies, making them more successful while also attending to the patient's overall well-being.

The idea that integrative therapies are unsupported by science is another misconception. In actuality, a large number of complementary medicines used in integrative oncology have undergone extensive testing and are backed by data attesting to their effectiveness and safety. As a result of continuous study, the area is always changing, and conventional cancer care regimens are increasingly incorporating integrative approaches.

The idea that integrative medicine is a one-size-fits-all strategy must be debunked. Integrative oncology's customized approach allows for the customization of treatments to meet the unique requirements and preferences of every patient. With this tailored approach, integrative therapies are safely incorporated into a thorough, scientifically supported cancer care plan.

Integrative oncology is a patient-focused, all-encompassing approach to cancer treatment that blends the finest aspects of complementary and conventional medicine. Beyond just treating symptoms, the advantages cover a wide range of facets related to a patient's overall health. Healthcare professionals and patients can collaborate to optimize cancer treatment outcomes and improve overall quality of life by clearing up common misconceptions and embracing the evidence-based concepts of integrative medicine.

CHAPTER FIVE

DIETARY METHODS

NUTRITION'S ROLE IN CANCER TREATMENT AND PREVENTION

A well-balanced, nutrient-rich diet is essential for maintaining general health because it plays a critical role in cancer prevention and therapy. Dietary decisions affect several variables, including oxidative stress, immunological response, and inflammation. The association between nutrition and cancer is complex. A healthy body is better able to resist the obstacles that cancer's onset and spread present.

The idea of anti-cancer diets has gained popularity in the field of cancer therapy and prevention. These diets place a strong emphasis on eating foods high in phytochemicals, antioxidants, and other bioactive substances that can stop the formation of cancer cells. For example, the Mediterranean diet is frequently advised because of its focus on fruits, vegetables, whole grains, and healthy fats; this represents a comprehensive approach to nutrition that is consistent with methods for preventing cancer.

VITAMINS AND SUPPLEMENTS IN CANCER CARE

Vitamins and supplements are also very important in the treatment of cancer. Even while eating a balanced diet is important, some nutritional supplements can help with conventional cancer treatments.

For example, research has shown that vitamin D may lower the risk of several malignancies, thus supplementing with it may help those who are deficient. Supplements should be used carefully though, as taking too many of them could have unexpected effects.

Determining the right supplementation for each patient requires a customized strategy under the direction of medical professionals.

Anti-cancer diets frequently highlight particular food groups and their possible effects on the prevention and treatment of cancer. Broccoli and cauliflower are examples of cruciferous vegetables, which are noted for having high concentrations of sulforaphane, an anti-cancer chemical. Antioxidant-rich berries are also frequently advised because of their ability to reduce inflammation and oxidative stress. Furthermore, adding omega-3 fatty acids to foods like fatty fish has been linked to anti-cancer benefits.

When it comes to cancer treatment, nutrition is essential for helping patients get through treatments like radiation and chemotherapy. During the difficult course of treatment, a healthy diet can strengthen the immune system, reduce side effects, and improve general well-being. It is essential to maintain a healthy weight through eating since malnourishment or extreme weight loss might impair the body's capacity to heal and tolerate treatment.

It is impossible to exaggerate the role that nutrition plays in both preventing and treating cancer. Nutrient-dense meals, vitamins, and supplements are the mainstays of anti-cancer diets, which provide a comprehensive strategy to aid the body's defense against cancer. Personalized dietary strategies are being incorporated into cancer care plans, which emphasizes how important it is to take into account each patient's unique health profile and treatment plan to maximize outcomes for cancer patients.

CHAPTER SIX

MIND-BODY METHODS

STRESS REDUCTION AND CANCER

In the field of mind-body approaches, there has been a lot of discussion on the complex relationship between stress reduction and cancer. According to research, long-term stress may hurt an individual's general health as well as accelerate the development of cancer. Stress-reduction strategies including deep breathing, guided visualization, and relaxation exercises are now essential parts of complementary cancer care. By reducing the physiological and psychological impacts of stress, these methods hope to create a more conducive environment for the body's natural healing mechanisms.

MEDITATION AND MINDFULNESS

These two disciplines have become well-known for their ability to support the mental and emotional health of cancer patients. Focused concentration and increased awareness are hallmarks of meditation, which provides a haven for people to work through the challenges of their condition. On the other hand, mindfulness promotes an accepting and peaceful presence in the present moment while avoiding judgment. These methods show promise for strengthening the immune system and improving general quality of life, in addition to easing the psychological toll that comes with cancer.

YOGA AND CANCER CARE

Because yoga takes a comprehensive approach to mental and physical health, it has become more and more fashionable to incorporate yoga into cancer care. Yoga offers a complete mind-body experience by combining physical postures, breath control, and meditation. Research indicates that yoga may help lessen the symptoms of cancer, such as anxiety, weariness, and insomnia. Furthermore, because some yoga poses are gentle, even that receiving cancer treatment can access them, giving them a helpful way to exercise and decompress.

ART AND MUSIC THERAPY

These forms of expressive and creative healing have become popular choices for those facing cancer. These therapeutic approaches acknowledge the powerful influence of artistic expression on the resolution of emotional wounds. Through the use of various artistic mediums, art therapy allows people to explore and share their feelings, leading to self-discovery and the development of coping skills. In contrast, music therapy makes use of music's transforming potential to improve emotional well-being, lessen anxiety, and ease pain. Both approaches provide special means for people to work with and manage the range of emotions that come with receiving a cancer diagnosis, encouraging self-expression and empowerment.

The use of mind-body methods in cancer treatment is a comprehensive strategy that acknowledges the relationship between mental and physical health. A more complete support network for those coping with cancer is provided via stress-reduction techniques, yoga, meditation, art, and music therapy, which provide pathways to recovery, resiliency, and enhanced quality of life.

CHAPTER SEVEN

ALTERNATIVE MEDICINE

BOTH ACUPRESSURE AND ACUPUNCTURE

Traditional Chinese medicine practices like acupuncture and acupressure involve stimulating particular body sites to balance Qi or energy flow, and aid in healing. Acupressure applies pressure on these points with the hands, fingers, or other utensils; acupuncture uses tiny needles put into these sites. The foundation of both modalities is the idea of meridians, which are energy channels that permit Qi to move.

The fundamental tenet of acupuncture and acupressure is that a variety of health problems can arise from imbalances or obstructions in the movement of Qi. These treatments work to relieve pain, regulate energy, and enhance general health by stimulating or pressing on particular places. Acupressure is a non-invasive option that is appropriate for people who may be allergic to needles, whereas acupuncture requires the insertion of needles into the skin.

MASSAGE THERAPY

The goal of massage therapy, a popular alternative therapy, is to improve health and well-being by manipulating the body's soft tissues. Different areas of physical and mental wellness are targeted by different massage techniques, including Swedish massage, deep tissue massage, and reflexology. Reduction of tension, alleviation of pain, increased relaxation, and improved circulation are some advantages of massage treatment.

The physical manipulation of muscles and tissues to induce blood flow and relieve tension are the mechanics underlying massage treatment. Furthermore, the body's natural feel-good chemicals called endorphins can be released as a result of the tactile stimulation that occurs during a massage. Apart from its physiological advantages, massage therapy also attends to psychological well-being, providing a comprehensive approach to health that takes into account the mind and body.

ONCOLOGY HERBAL MEDICINE

For ages, herbal medicine has been an essential component of conventional medical systems, and its use as a supplemental therapy in oncology is becoming more widely acknowledged. Using materials derived from plants to support cancer patients during treatment and control adverse effects is known as herbal medicine in oncology. Certain herbs, like mistletoe, green tea, and turmeric, have demonstrated potential in the treatment of cancer.

These herbal medicines' ability to reduce inflammation, promote immunity, and provide antioxidants makes them popular choices. Herbal medicine is seen as a supplemental strategy that may help reduce symptoms, enhance quality of life, and improve general well-being, even while it is not a replacement for traditional cancer therapies like chemotherapy and radiation therapy. Before using herbal medication, patients receiving cancer treatment should speak with their healthcare provider to be sure it will work with their particular treatment plan and to avoid any potential interactions.

CHAPTER EIGHT

CHANGES IN LIFESTYLE

EXERCISE AND PHYSICAL ACTIVITY

Maintaining a healthy lifestyle requires regular exercise and physical activity. Physical activity improves general well-being in addition to aiding with weight management. Exercise has a well-established ability to lower the risk of several chronic illnesses, including diabetes, obesity, and heart disease. Regular exercise is also proven to improve mood and lower stress and anxiety levels, which in turn improve mental health.

Furthermore, a robust and functional musculoskeletal system depends on exercise. Weight-bearing activities, like jogging, weight training, and walking, support healthy bones and can help stave off diseases like osteoporosis. Strength training and aerobic exercise regimens together can improve a person's physical and mental well-being over the long run.

CANCER AND SLEEP

In recent times, there has been a growing focus on the correlation between cancer and sleep. Sleep disturbances have been linked to an increased risk of cancer. Getting enough good sleep is essential for general health and well-being. Certain types of cancer may develop as a result of abnormal sleep habits, which include getting too little or poor quality sleep.

The sleep-wake cycle controls the body's circadian rhythm, which affects several physiological functions, such as the immune system and cell repair. These activities may be hampered by disturbances to this normal cycle, such as those brought on by erratic sleep schedules or working night shifts, which may encourage the growth of cancer cells. Thus, promoting general health and lowering the risk of cancer require prioritizing excellent sleep hygiene, setting up a regular sleep routine, and providing a comfortable sleeping environment.

CESSATION OF SMOKING

One of the most effective lifestyle changes one can undertake to enhance health and fend off diseases is to give up smoking. Smoking is associated with numerous health concerns, such as respiratory disorders, cardiovascular illnesses, and cancer, and it is one of the primary preventable causes of mortality globally. The advantages of stopping smoking become apparent very quickly, as lung capacity, cardiovascular health, and general respiratory health all improve.

Apart from the short-term health advantages, stopping smoking also dramatically lowers the long-term chance of acquiring illnesses that could be fatal. Because of the body's remarkable capacity for healing, people who stop smoking can reduce their risk of heart disease, stroke, and several malignancies. The road to quitting smoking can be aided by supportive tools like counseling, medication, and nicotine replacement therapy, which can turn it into a life-changing move toward healthy living.

ALCOHOL CONSUMPTION

A healthy lifestyle revolves around using alcohol in moderation. Excessive or binge drinking can have negative impacts on one's physical and emotional well-being, even if other research indicates that moderate alcohol consumption may have some health benefits. Long-term alcohol misuse is associated with heart problems, liver disease, and a higher chance of developing several types of cancer.

Minimizing health hazards requires understanding and following suggested alcohol intake guidelines. Commonly speaking, these recommendations support moderate drinking, which is commonly understood to mean no more than one drink for women and two for men each day. It's crucial to remember that everyone reacts differently to alcohol, and some people may be more vulnerable to the harmful consequences of even moderate alcohol consumption.

CHAPTER NINE

COMPREHENSIVE METHODS FOR PARTICULAR CANCERS

BREAST CANCER

To address the various facets of this illness, integrative techniques for breast cancer comprise a thorough plan that blends alternative therapies with traditional medical treatments. While radiation, chemotherapy, and surgery are still the main forms of treatment, integrative methods place a strong emphasis on dietary changes, mind-body practices, and lifestyle adjustments.

Integrative oncology promotes regular physical activity and a nutritious diet full of foods high in anti-inflammatory components for its patients. In addition, complementary therapies like massage and acupuncture work to promote general well-being by reducing adverse effects associated with treatment.

CANCER OF THE PROSTATE

Prostate cancer-specific integrative techniques take a multifaceted approach to addressing the particular problems this cancer presents. Integrative care emphasizes dietary adjustments and physical activity in addition to standard therapies including radiation, surgery, and hormone therapy. Patients with prostate cancer may find it helpful to include particular nutrients and supplements that have been proven to enhance prostate health. Meditation and yoga are examples of mind-body techniques that can help manage stress and improve quality of life both during and after treatment.

LUNG CANCER

Recognizing the complexities of lung cancer, the integrative care paradigm mixes complementary therapies with standard treatments like chemotherapy, surgery, and targeted medicines. Dietary modifications and nutritional support are essential, with an emphasis on foods that strengthen the immune system and reduce inflammation. Exercise and breathing exercises are part of pulmonary rehabilitation, which helps to improve lung function and general physical health. The emotional toll that lung cancer and its treatment take on patients may be lessened with the use of mindfulness-based stress reduction and counseling.

COLORECTAL CANCER

Integrative therapy methods for colorectal cancer acknowledge the value of a holistic approach to care. While surgery, chemotherapy, and radiation therapy continue to be crucial, lifestyle adjustments including eating differently, working out frequently, and controlling weight all play a big part. The practice of integrative oncology advocates for a plant-based, high-fiber diet since it has been linked to a decreased risk of colon cancer recurrence. Acupuncture and herbal supplements are examples of complementary therapies that are investigated to help patients manage the adverse effects of treatment and improve their general health.

BLOOD CANCERS: LYMPHOMA AND LEUKAEMIA

Leukemia and lymphoma are two blood malignancies that require specialized care that takes into account their particular characteristics. Integrative techniques emphasize immune system support and treatment side effect management, but conventional treatments including radiation, chemotherapy, and stem cell transplantation are essential components. Supplements and dietary changes are examples of nutritional therapies that try to improve immune function and lessen the effects of chemotherapy. For those with blood malignancies, mind-body techniques like guided imagery and meditation may help lower stress and enhance their general quality of life. To meet the many requirements of patients during their cancer journey, integrative approaches acknowledge the synergy between conventional and complementary therapy.

CHAPTER TEN

LIFE SPAN AND LIFE QUALITY

LIFE AFTER CANCER TREATMENT

For those who have finished their cancer treatment, the journey of survival commences. This stage is frequently characterized by a mix of accomplishment, hope, and relief. But returning to a "normal" life following cancer treatment can provide its own set of difficulties.

Those who have survived may struggle with emotional trauma, bodily alterations, and recurrence anxiety. Rebuilding one's life after cancer requires taking into account not just the physical but also the emotional and social components of healing.

Friends, family, and programs for survivorship are examples of support networks that are vital in assisting people in navigating the unknowns of life after cancer.

Chemotherapy, radiation, and surgery can have long-term side effects that survivors must deal with. These adverse impacts might differ greatly and impact several facets of an individual's life, such as overall well-being, cognitive abilities, and physical health. To effectively control these long-term negative effects, a comprehensive strategy must be implemented. This could entail continuing medical supervision, therapy plans, and lifestyle modifications.

Furthermore, survivors and healthcare professionals need to collaborate to create individualized care plans that address certain long-term issues. Putting a strong emphasis on prevention and continuing to take a proactive approach to healthcare can greatly improve the quality of life for cancer survivors who are experiencing long-lasting side effects.

EMOTIONAL AND PSYCHOLOGICAL WELL-BEING

Receiving a cancer diagnosis has a significant emotional and psychological impact that lasts long after treatment is finished. To cope with the aftermath of cancer, one must handle a variety of emotions, such as fear, worry, and occasionally even post-traumatic stress disorder. During this stage, getting help from loved ones, support groups, and mental health specialists becomes crucial. Adopting techniques like social support, therapy, and mindfulness can assist survivors in navigating the emotional landscape and building resilience. Fostering emotional and psychological well-being requires adopting self-care techniques and cultivating an optimistic outlook. Furthermore, acknowledging the value of candid communication and ending the taboo around mental health concerns in survivorship helps to foster a community that is accepting and encouraging.

Life following cancer treatment is a complex path that goes beyond physical healing. A comprehensive and customized strategy is needed to manage long-term side effects, taking into account the particular difficulties that each survivor may encounter. Making emotional and psychological health a priority is essential for building resilience and assisting people in regaining a sense of normalcy and purpose in their lives following the life-altering experience of cancer treatment.

CHAPTER ELEVEN

COMBINING TRADITIONAL AND ALTERNATIVE MEDICAL PRACTICES

COOPERATION AMONG HEALTHCARE PRACTITIONERS

Within the field of medicine, the amalgamation of conventional and integrative medicine underscores the significance of interdisciplinary collaboration among medical practitioners. With its foundation in cutting-edge technologies and evidence-based methods, conventional medicine seeks to blend its strengths with integrative medicine's patient-centered, holistic approach. To develop thorough and individualized treatment plans for patients, doctors, nurses, therapists, and other healthcare professionals frequently collaborate in this way.

The practitioners' sharing of information and experience is a crucial component of this partnership. While integrative medicine practitioners offer insights into complementary therapies, lifestyle interventions, and mind-body practices, conventional medical doctors add a wealth of scientific expertise and clinical experience. Through the promotion of transparent communication and reciprocal regard, this cooperative model aims to leverage the advantages of both strategies to deliver more comprehensive and efficient patient care.

OPPORTUNITIES AND DIFFICULTIES

There are difficulties in integrating integrative and conventional medicine. The two techniques' different therapeutic paradigms and philosophies present a major barrier. It takes dedication to comprehend and honor one another's viewpoints to close these differences. Furthermore, problems with insurance reimbursement, legal frameworks, and standard operating procedures might make it difficult to apply integrative approaches in traditional healthcare settings.

Notwithstanding these obstacles, there exist noteworthy prospects for enhancing patient outcomes and the provision of healthcare services. The principles of integrative medicine include patient-centered care, prevention, and the connection between mental, emotional, and physical health. Integrative medicine can improve the efficacy of conventional therapies and contribute to a more comprehensive and holistic healthcare system by treating the underlying causes of health conditions and incorporating lifestyle improvements.

PATIENT EMPOWERMENT AND EDUCATION

Patient empowerment and education play a key part in the effective combination of conventional and integrative care. Patients who are knowledgeable and involved are better able to take charge of their health and actively participate in healthcare decisions. While integrative medicine places a strong emphasis on teaching patients about lifestyle variables, self-care techniques, and complementary medicines, conventional medicine frequently excels at giving evidence-based information.

 Building a cooperative relationship between patients and healthcare professionals is essential to empowering patients. This can entail offering tools, teaching materials, and guidance on changing one's way of life. The intention is to establish a healthcare setting where individuals are empowered to make decisions that are consistent with their values and preferences. The transition to patient-centered care has been shown to increase overall patient satisfaction and well-being in addition to improving treatment adherence.

Successful cooperation between medical experts, overcoming obstacles seizing opportunities, and putting a high priority on patient education and empowerment are all necessary for the merger of conventional and integrative medicine.